KETO

MW01015931

SLOW COOKER

RECIPES

*Quick and Easy, Low-Carb Keto
Diet Crock Pot Recipes for Weight
Loss and a Healthier You*

Heather Somers

DISCLAIMER

TABLE OF CONTENTS

INTRODUCTION

Living the ketogenic lifestyle is all about eating delicious, healthy whole foods that keep carb counts low and energy high as we sculpt our bodies and minds to perfection. And now there is even better news for those of us trying to maintain our ketogenic eating habits while maintaining a go-go-go lifestyle – the slow cooker.

Yes, the slow cooker was likely responsible for some of the delicious carb-rich meals grandma used to whip up, and that is part of the reason many low-carb cooks stay away from slow cooking. However, the slow cooker is experiencing a revival thanks to busy but carb-conscious cooks. That's where this book comes in.

The Ketogenic Slow Cooker Recipes cookbook contains delicious recipes that take 20 minutes or less to prepare before you put it in the slow cooker. The recipes contain, for the most part, short, simple lists of ingredients. All of this means you can toss your ingredients into the slow cooker in the morning and have a home-cooked ketogenic-friendly meal waiting for you in the evening.

Most importantly, **each of the recipes contains 8 grams or less of carbs per serving**, and that will ensure your body maintains its ketogenic balance. The recipes provided take you from morning to night with delicious breakfast options like Crimini, Sausage and Cheese Strata, and a delicious take on oatmeal without any of the actual carb-rich oatmeal.

Meal options include delicious versions of your cozy favourites like Meaty Cauliflower Lasagna and BLT Chicken Salad, or elegant dishes like our Fig and Goat-Cheese Stuffed Chicken or Braised Pork Belly.

If you're hosting a party or simply inviting a few friends over, you can rest assured your appetizers are being whipped up in your slow cooker as you attend to your other errands. The appetizer selection includes lovely Portabella Pizza Bites, Creamy Asiago Spinach Dip, and a beautiful Asparagus Bacon Bouquet.

The delicious, low-carb meals created for you in the Ketogenic Slow Cooker Recipes cookbook makes it even easier to stick to your ketogenic plan and ensures your road to health, beauty, and wellness is a smooth and delicious one.

WHAT IS THE KETOGENIC DIET?

The ketogenic diet provides you with a chance to transform your body into a fat-fighting machine while eating foods that you love. The key to following the diet is turning everything you thought you knew about food on its head.

For decades we have heard about the evils of fat and why decreasing fat in the diet leads to improved health and a reduction in weight. It turns out, however, that fat, is not the enemy, and in fact, on the ketogenic diet, fat is one of your closest friends. In fact, it is fat that you're going to turn to as your trusted energy source when it comes to meal times, snack time, or anytime.

Food provides us with essential energy to keep our bodies functioning. When you take a bite of food your body jumps into action. The carbohydrates in food are converted into glucose which is used as energy. However, when the consumption of carbohydrates is significantly reduced, the body starts to use fat for energy instead. This process is called ketosis. Once your body goes into ketosis, you begin to burn up the stored fats as well as the fats you ingest, and this in turn leads to significant weight loss.

The ketogenic diet that we know today was initially developed by Dr. Russel Wilder in the 1920s as a treatment for epilepsy. Further research into the diet also revealed that the ratio of carbs to fats to proteins also produced significant weight loss in patients. The diet was further developed by the creation of a formula that more precisely described the amount of fats to carbohydrates to proteins a patient should consume in order to trigger ketosis. The original formula relies on the consumption of less than 15 g of calories per day from carbohydrates, with the remaining calories coming from fat and to a lesser extent from protein.

As an epileptic treatment, the ketogenic diet proved successful. However, it later became better known for a plethora of other health benefits not linked to the initial treatment. In addition to the significant weight loss that occurs as a result of going into a state of ketosis, patients have reported improved memory and alertness as well as better sleep patterns. Additionally, the ketogenic diet has been used as a tool to target fat in the abdomen which is particularly dangerous. Eating the right composition of carbs, proteins, and fats has also been shown to decrease triglycerides in the blood and balance insulin levels. The change in the types of foods consumed ultimately decreases bad fats and increases good, heart-healthy fats in the system.

Overall, the ketogenic diet has proven to be a great choice for better physical and mental health. It is important to note, however, that the diet relies heavily on the right balance of macronutrients, carbohydrates, fat, and protein, which is why it is essential to consult a medical professional before beginning your ketogenic lifestyle journey.

BREAKFAST RECIPES

Crimini Sausage and Cheese Strata

Serves: 4

Preparation time: 15 minutes

Cooking time: 3 hours and 45 minutes

Ingredients:

20 Crimini mushrooms

2 Italian sausage links

½ cup Mozzarella, shredded

2 tbsp heavy cream

¼ cup low-sodium chicken stock

1 tsp oregano

2 tsp salt

1 tsp black pepper

2 tbsp ghee

extra virgin olive oil

Directions:

1. Lightly coat slow cooker with olive oil.
2. Mix heavy cream with chicken stock, set aside.
3. Quarter mushrooms and toss with 1 tsp salt and oregano, place in bottom of slow cooker.

4. Slice sausage into ½" discs, and place on mushrooms, pour chicken stock mix on top.
5. Sprinkle with cheese, and cook in slow cooker on high for 3.5 hours.

Nutrition (per serving)

Calories 140

Carbs 4.9

Fat 10

Protein 8

Sodium 1318 (mg)

Sugar 2

The New York Meat Bagel

Serves: 4

Preparation time: 15 minutes

Cooking time: 4 hours

Ingredients:

1 lb ground beef

1 tbsp almond flour

1 tbsp black pepper

2 tbsp coconut milk

1 tsp salt

Extra virgin olive oil

Topping

3 slices cheddar cheese

1 tomato, sliced

1 cup lettuce, chopped

Directions:

1. Lightly coat a 6 qt. slow cooker with extra virgin olive oil.
2. Combine beef, salt, black pepper, coconut milk, almond flour in bowl.
3. Divide into 6 equal portions, and shape each one into a ½" thick circle.

4. Using a bottle cap, cut out the center of each circle so you have six bagel-shaped circles.

5. Place meat bagel halves in slow cooker, cover, and cook on medium for 4 hours.

6. Once done, remove from slow cooker, toast in toaster oven for a crispier bagel if desired, and top with lettuce, tomato, and cheese.

Nutrition (per serving)

Calories 499

Carbs 5 g

Fat 28 g

Protein 55 g

Sodium 1055 mg

Sugar 1 g

Ham and Zucchini Quiche

Serves: 4

Preparation time: 15 minutes

Cooking time: 5 hours

Ingredients:

2 zucchini, peeled

4 x 1oz slices Picnic Ham

4 eggs

1 tsp salt

1 tsp black pepper

Extra virgin olive oil

Directions:

1. Brush your slow cooker with extra virgin olive oil.
2. Whisk eggs, set aside.
3. Slice zucchini into ½" discs and sprinkle with salt, black pepper.
4. Place half the zucchini slices on bottom of slow cooker, layer ham slices on top, pour eggs over ham.
5. Place remaining zucchini on top, and cook on medium for 5 hours.

Nutrition per serving:

Calories 278

Carbs 24 g

Fat 18 g

Protein 5

Sodium 605 mg

Sugar 2 g

Rainbow Pepper Breakfast Casserole

Serves: 4

Preparation time: 15 minutes

Cooking time: 8 hours

Ingredients:

½ red bell pepper, diced

½ green bell pepper, diced

½ yellow bell pepper, diced

½ cup almond milk

1 cup artichoke hearts, frozen or fresh, quartered

8 eggs

1 tsp oregano

1 tsp black pepper

1 tsp salt

Extra virgin olive oil

Directions:

1. Lightly coat slow cooker with extra virgin olive oil
2. Whip up eggs, add remaining ingredients, save artichoke hearts.
3. Coat slow cooker with olive oil.
4. Place artichoke hearts in slow cooker, pour egg mixture over top.
5. Cook for 8 hours on low.

Nutrition per serving:

Calories 177

Carbs 4.8 g

Fat 12 g

Protein 12 g

Sodium 709 mg

Sugar 3 g

Nutty Oatless Oatmeal

Serves: 5

Preparation time: 15 minutes

Cooking time: 7 hours

Ingredients:

¼ cup flaxseed

¼ cup almonds, chopped

¼ cup walnuts, chopped

1 cup coconut milk

1 cup water

1 tsp almond butter

1 tsp cardamom seeds

1 tsp ghee

Directions:

1. Coat slow cooker with ghee.
2. Mix ingredients together, and pour into slow cooker
3. Cook on low for 7 hours.

Nutrition per serving:

Calories 266

Carbs 5.2 g

Fat 20 g

Protein 5 g

Sodium 9 mg

Sugar 2 g

Spinach Quiche

Serves: 4

Preparation time: 15 minutes

Cooking time: 7 hours

Ingredients:

8 eggs

1 cup spinach, chopped

1 tbsp coconut flour

¾ cup walnuts

1/3 cup sunflower seeds

1 onion, diced

½ cup Mozzarella, shredded

½ tsp black pepper

½ tsp salt

Extra virgin olive oil

Directions:

1. Place walnuts, sunflower seeds in food processor with ghee, and blend until crumbly.
2. Lightly coat slow cooker with a little olive oil, and press walnut mixture into bottom of slow cooker.
3. Heat 2 tbsp olive oil in skillet, add onion, and sauté for a minute, and remove from heat.
4. Add spinach, salt, black pepper. Mix and remove from heat.

5. Spoon spinach mixture onto crust in slow cooker.

6. Whisk eggs with 2 tbsp olive oil and coconut flour, pour over spinach, and top with grated cheese.

7. Cook on low for 7 hours.

Nutrition per serving:

Calories 297

Carbs 5.6 g

Fat 22 g

Protein 19 g

Sodium 418 mg

Sugar 2 g

APPETIZER RECIPES

Asparagus Bacon Bouquet

Serves: 4

Preparation time: 10 minutes

Cooking time: 4 hours

Ingredients:

8 asparagus spears, trimmed

8 slices bacon

1 tsp black pepper

Extra virgin olive oil

Directions:

1. Coat slow cooker with extra virgin olive oil.
2. Slice spears in half, and sprinkle with black pepper
3. Wrap three spear halves with one slice bacon, and set inside slow cooker.
4. Cook for 4 hours on medium.

Nutrition per serving:

Calories 345

Carbs 2 g

Fat 27 g

Protein 22 g

Sodium 1311 mg

Sugar 0 g

Creamy Asiago Spinach Dip

Serves: 6

Preparation time: 15 minutes

Cooking time: 4 hours

Ingredients:

6 cups spinach, wash, chopped

½ cup artichoke hearts

½ cup cream cheese

½ cup Asiago cheese, grated

½ cup almond milk

1 tsp black pepper

Extra virgin olive oil

Directions:

1. Coat slow cooker with olive oil.
2. Place cream cheese and almond milk in blender, and mix until smooth.
3. Finely chop spinach, add to blender along with salt and black pepper, and mix.
4. Place spinach mixture in blender, add artichoke hearts, and mix in with a spatula.
5. Sprinkle Asiago cheese on top, and cook on medium for 4 hours.
6. Serve dip with a selection of veggies like broccoli florets and carrot sticks.

Nutrition per serving:

Calories 214

Carbs 4 g

Fat 19 g

Protein 8 g

Sodium 380 mg

Sugar 1 g

Madras Curry Chicken Bites

Serves: 4

Preparation time: 10 minutes

Cooking time: 7 hours

Ingredients:

1 lb chicken breasts, skinless, boneless

4 cloves garlic, grated

1 tsp ginger, grated

2 cups low-sodium chicken stock

2 lemons, juiced

1 tsp coriander, crushed

1 tsp cumin

½ tsp fenugreek

1 tbsp curry powder

½ tsp cinnamon

1½ tsp salt

1 tsp black pepper

Extra virgin olive oil

Directions:

1. Cube chicken breast into ½" pieces, and sprinkle with ½ tsp salt and ½ tsp black pepper.
2. Heat 3 tbsp extra virgin olive oil in skillet, add chicken breasts, and brown.

3. Place chicken breasts in slow cooker.

4. Add chicken stock, garlic, lemon juice, spices, and salt.

5. Cook on low for 7 hours.

Nutrition per serving:

Calories 234

Carbs 3 g

Fat 8 g

Protein 38 g

Sodium 782 mg

Sugar 0 g

Spiced Jicama Wedges with Cilantro Chutney

Serves: 8

Preparation time: 15 minutes

Cooking time: 4 hours

Ingredients:

1 lb jicama, peeled

1 tsp paprika

½ tsp dried parsley

2 tsp salt

2 tsp black pepper

Extra virgin olive oil

Cilantro Chutney

1 tsp dill chopped

¼ cup cilantro

½ tsp salt

1 tsp paprika

1tsp black pepper

2 lemons, juiced

¼ cup extra virgin olive oil

Directions:

1. Slice jicama into 1" wedges, and submerge in a bowl of cold water for 20 minutes.

2. Place paprika, oregano, salt, black pepper in a bowl, and toss with jicama.
3. Add 5 tbsp extra virgin olive oil into bowl, and coat well.
4. Place jicama in slow cooker, and cook on high for 4 hours.
5. Combine ingredients for chutney in blender, mix, and refrigerate until jicama wedges are ready to serve.

Nutrition per serving:

Calories 94

Carbs 5.2 g

Fat 8 g

Protein 1 g

Sodium 879 mg

Sugar 1 g

Teriyaki Chicken Wings

Serves: 4

Preparation time: 10 minutes

Cooking time: 4 hours minutes

Ingredients

2 lb chicken wings

2 tsp ginger, grated

4 cloves garlic, grated

¼ cup soy sauce

4 dates, pitted

Extra virgin olive oil

Directions

1. Place dates in food processor along with 2 tbsp soy sauce, and mix until pasty.
2. Combine ginger, garlic, soy sauce, and dates in bowl, add chicken wings, coat, and refrigerate overnight.
3. Coat slow cooker with a little sesame oil, add chicken wings, and cook on high for 4 hours.

Nutrition per serving:

Calories 354

Carbs 5.5 g

Fat 16 g

Protein 45 g

Sodium 730 mg

Sugar 0 g

Portabella Pizza Bites

Serves: 8

Preparation time: 15 minutes

Cooking time: 5 hours

Ingredients:

8 Portabella Mushrooms

½ lb ground pork

1 medium onion, diced

4 cloves garlic, grated

2 cups crushed tomato

½ cup Mozzarella, shredded

¼ cup Parmesan

½ tsp oregano

1 tsp salt

1 tsp black pepper

Garnish

½ cup parsley, chopped

Directions:

1. Coat 6 qt. slow cooker with extra virgin olive oil
2. Heat 3 tbsp extra virgin olive oil in skillet, add pork, brown.
3. Mix crushed tomato with salt, black pepper, oregano, parmesan, and garlic.

4. Spoon a little tomato-parmesan mixture into each mushroom, add a little ground pork, and sprinkle with Mozzarella.
5. Place each mushroom in slow cooker (when layering do not put one mushroom directly on top of the other, instead straddle one mushroom on two).
6. Cook pizza bites on medium for 5 hours.
7. Sprinkle a little parsley on top before serving.

Nutrition per serving:

Calories 106

Carbs 5.6 g

Fat 3 g

Protein 13 g

Sodium 421 mg

Sugar 2 g

SOUP RECIPES

Creamy Coconut Butternut Squash Soup

Serves: 8

Preparation time: 15 minutes

Cooking time: 5 hours

Ingredients:

1 acorn squash

1 bell pepper, seeded, diced

2 carrots, sliced

1 onion, diced

2 tbsp ginger, grated

1 cup coconut cream

2 cups low-sodium chicken broth

1 tsp paprika

1 tsp salt

Extra virgin olive oil

Directions:

1. Slice squash in half, peel, remove seeds, and flesh.

2. Chop squash into cubes, and place into slow cooker.

3. Place 4 tbsp extra virgin olive oil in skillet, add onion, ginger, sauté for a minute.
4. Add coconut milk, onion, ginger, carrot, red bell pepper, paprika, and salt into slow cooker.
5. Cook soup on medium for 5 hours.
6. In cooker use hand immersion blender to blend until creamy.

Nutrition per serving:

Calories 140

Carbs 8.7 g

Fat 11 g

Protein 2 g

Sodium 315 mg

Sugar 1 g

Popeye's Turkey Soup

Serves: 8

Preparation time: 15 minutes

Cooking time: 4 hours

Ingredients:

1 turkey breast (2.5 lbs)

6 cups spinach, chopped

1 medium onion, diced.

4 garlic cloves, grated

2 cups low-sodium chicken stock

1 tsp rosemary

½ tsp thyme

1 tsp salt

1 tsp black pepper

Extra virgin olive oil

Directions:

1. Brush slow cooker with extra virgin olive oil and set slow cooker to medium.
2. Slice turkey breast into ½" cubes.
3. Heat 4 tbsp extra virgin olive oil in skillet, add turkey breast and brown.
4. Place turkey breast in slow cooker along with spinach, onion, garlic, chicken stock, rosemary, thyme, salt and black pepper, mix and cover.

5. Cook on medium for 4 hours.

Nutrition per serving:

Calories 193

Carbs 8.8 g

Fat 6 g

Protein 25 g

Sodium 1781 mg

Sugar 0 g

White Chicken Chili

Serves: 6

Preparation time: 15 minutes

Cooking time: 7 hours

Ingredients:

1 lb ground chicken

2 tomatoes, chopped

1 green bell pepper, seeded, diced

1 medium onion, diced

4 cloves garlic, grated

2 tbsp tomato paste

1 tsp oregano

1 tsp cumin

1 tsp salt

1 tsp black pepper

Extra virgin olive oil

Directions:

1. Brush slow cooker with extra virgin olive oil, and set slow cooker on high.
2. Heat 4 tbsp extra virgin olive oil in skillet, add ground chicken, and brown.
3. Add onion, garlic, into chicken and sauté for 30 seconds, place mixture in slow cooker.

4. Add tomatoes, oregano, cumin, salt, black pepper into slow cooker.

5. Cook on low for 7 hours.

Nutrition per serving:

Calories 161

Carbs 5 g

Fat 8 g

Protein 17 g

Sodium 346 mg

Sugar 2 g

Silky Broccoli and Cheese Soup

Serves: 8

Preparation Time: 10 minutes

Cooking Time: 3 hours

Ingredients:

3 cups broccoli florets

½ cup cashews, soaked overnight, chopped

½ cup cheddar, grated

2 cups low-sodium chicken stock

1 cup coconut cream

1 tsp coconut flour

1 tsp salt

1 tsp black pepper

Extra virgin olive oil

4 tbsp ghee

Directions:

1. Heat ghee in skillet over medium heat.
2. Mix coconut flour into skillet quickly.
3. Add coconut cream, mix until smooth, and set aside.
4. Brush slow cooker with extra virgin olive oil, and set on high.

5. Place broccoli in slow cooker with chicken stock, salt, black pepper, cashews. Mix and cover for 10 minutes.

6. Stir in coconut cream mixture and cheese, and cook for 3 hours.

Nutrition per serving:

Calories 216

Carbs 7 g

Fat 20 g

Protein 5 g

Sodium 386 mg

Sugar 0 g

SIDE DISH RECIPES

Parmesan Garlic Mustard Greens

Serves: 4

Preparation time: 5 minutes

Cooking time: 3 hours

Ingredients:

4 cups Mustard Greens

4 cloves garlic, minced

¼ cup Parmesan

1/3 cup almonds

1 tsp salt

Extra virgin olive oil

Directions:

1. Chop mustard greens, and toss with 3 tbsp extra virgin olive oil, salt, black pepper.
2. Place almonds in food processor and chop.
3. Place mustard greens in slow cooker and top with almonds and parmesan.
4. Cook on high for 3 hours.

Nutrition per serving:

Calories 140

Carbs 4.9 g

Fat 11 g

Protein 8 g

Sodium 728 mg

Sugar 1 g

Lemon Butter Radish with Vanilla Note

Serves: 4

Preparation time: 10 minutes

Cooking time: 4 hours

Ingredients:

20 radishes, stemmed

½ cup ghee

1 lemon, juiced

¼ tsp vanilla

Extra virgin olive oil

Directions:

1. Place ghee in saucepan, melt.
2. Remove ghee from heat, add lemon, vanilla, salt.
3. Add radish to ghee, coat.
4. Place radish in slow cooker and cook on low for 4 hours.

Nutrition per serving:

Calories 259

Carbs 1 g

Fat 29 g

Protein 0 g

Sodium 9 mg

Sugar 0 g

Cheesy Cauliflower Puree

Serves: 4

Preparation time: 15 minutes

Cooking time: 4 hours

Ingredients:

1 small head cauliflower

1 cup cheddar cheese

½ cup half-and-half cream

½ tsp nutmeg

½ tsp white pepper

1 tsp salt

Extra virgin olive oil

Directions:

1. Coat slow cooker with extra virgin olive oil.
2. Chop cauliflower into small florets, and place in slow cooker, add salt, black pepper, nutmeg, cream, and cheddar cheese. Mix.
3. Cook on medium for 4 hours.
4. Using hand immersion blender, mix until smooth.

Nutrition per serving:

Calories 202

Carbs 5.5 g

Fat 17 g

Protein 9 g

Sodium 789 mg

Sugar 0 g

Cauliflower Rice

Serves: 4

Preparation time: 15 minutes

Cooking time: 3 hours

Ingredients:

1 small head cauliflower

1 cup low-sodium chicken stock

4 tbsp ghee

1 tsp salt

Directions:

1. Separate cauliflower into florets, place in food processor, and chop into rice-like granules.
2. Place ghee in bottom of slow-cooker, turn cooker to medium, and allow ghee to melt.
3. Place cauli-rice in slow cooker, add salt, chicken stock, and mix.
4. Cook on medium for 3 hours.

Nutrition per serving:

Calories 130

Carbs 3.5 g

Fat 13 g

Protein 2 g

Sodium 635 mg

Sugar 0 g

Spicy Squash Noodles

Serves: 4

Preparation time: 15 minutes

Cooking time: 7 hours

Ingredients:

1 spaghetti squash

1 tsp red pepper flakes

1 tsp salt

1 lemon, juiced

Extra virgin olive oil

Directions:

1. Slice spaghetti squash in half and remove seeds.
2. Drizzle inside of squash with a little olive oil and place in slow cooker.
3. Cook squash for 7 hours on medium.
4. Remove from slow cooker, cool.
5. Once cooled, use fork to scrape out squash flesh noodles.
6. Toss noodles with salt, lemon juice, and red pepper flakes.

Nutrition per serving:

Calories 55

Carbs 5.5 g

Fat 4 g

Protein 1 g

Sodium 594 mg

Sugar 0 g

Warm Walnut Cabbage Salad

Serves: 4

Preparation time: 10 minutes

Cooking time: 3 hours

Ingredients:

3 cups cabbage, shredded

½ cup walnuts, chopped

¼ cup flaxseed

1 tsp salt

2 tsp black pepper

Extra virgin olive oil

Directions:

1. Brush slow cooker with olive oil.
2. Add cabbage, walnuts, flaxseed, salt, black pepper to slow cooker and cook on high for 3 hours.

Nutrition per serving:

Calories 107

Carbs 4 g

Fat 9 g

Protein 4 g

Sodium 395 mg

Sugar 0 g

MAIN DISH RECIPES

Lime Chicken with Savoy Cabbage

Serves: 4

Preparation time: 10 minutes

Cooking time: 7 hours

Ingredients:

8 chicken thighs, skinless

2 cups Savoy cabbage, chopped

1 stalk celery, diced

1 medium onion, diced

1 tbsp ginger, grated

2 limes

1 tsp salt

1 tsp black pepper

Extra virgin olive oil

Directions:

1. Place 4 tbsp extra virgin olive oil in slow cooker, spread around the bottom.
2. Slice lime into ½" thick circles.
3. Place chicken in bottom of slow cooker, and sprinkle with ½ tsp salt and ½ tsp black pepper.
4. Top with lime slices. On top of those, place celery and cabbage.

5. Pour in chicken stock, and cook on low for 7 hours.
6. Serve with Spicy Squash Noodles.

Nutrition per serving:

Calories 273

Carbs 5.7 g

Fat 12 g

Protein 34 g

Sodium 689 mg

Sugar 0 g

Middle Eastern Lamb Zucchini Casserole

Serves: 6

Preparation time: 20 minutes

Cooking time: 7 hours

Ingredients:

4 zucchinis, peeled

1 lb ground lamb

½ cup coconut cream

2 eggs

¼ cup Parmesan

½ tsp cinnamon

½ tsp cloves

½ tsp cumin

1 tsp salt

1 tsp black pepper

Extra virgin olive oil

Directions:

1. Using mandolin, thinly-slice zucchini lengthwise.
2. Heat 3 tbsp extra virgin olive oil in skillet. Add lamb, cinnamon, cloves, and cumin. Brown.
3. Combine coconut cream with egg, salt, and black pepper.

4. Coat slow cooker with olive oil, place ¼ of zucchini strips on bottom of slow cooker.
5. Next brush coconut cream mixture on zucchini.
6. Place another layer of zucchini and half the remaining coconut cream, top with lamb, another layer of zucchini, remaining coconut cream.
7. Cook on low for 7 hours.

Nutrition per serving:

Calories 203

Carbs 4.7 g

Fat 10 g

Protein 25 g

Sodium 479 mg

Sugar 0 g

Ginger Steak Broccoli

Serves: 4

Preparation time: 10 minutes

Cooking time: 4 hours

Ingredients:

1 lb sirloin steak

3 cups broccoli florets (frozen ok)

1 cup low-sodium beef stock

1 tbsp grated ginger

½ tsp thyme

1 tsp salt

1 tsp black pepper

Extra virgin olive oil

Directions:

1. Slice sirloin steak against grain into ½" wide strips.
2. Place 4 tbsp extra virgin olive oil in skillet, add steak, and brown for a minute each side.
3. Place steak, broccoli florets, along with ginger, beef stock, and soy sauce in slow cooker.
4. Cook on medium-high for 4 hours.
5. Enjoy alone or with cauliflower rice.

Nutrition per serving:

Calories 273

Carbs 6 g

Fat 11 g

Protein 37 g

Sodium 714 mg

Sugar 0 g

BLT Chicken Salad

Serves: 4

Preparation time: 20 minutes

Cooking time: 4 hours

Ingredients:

4 x 4oz chicken breast

2 cup low-sodium chicken broth

8 slices bacon

2 cups romaine lettuce

1 tomato, diced

1 tsp salt

1 tsp black pepper

¼ cup organic mayonnaise

Extra virgin olive oil

Directions:

1. Coat slow cooker with a little olive oil, and set on high.
2. Tenderize chicken breast, and sprinkle each chicken breast with salt and black pepper.
3. Wrap each chicken breast with bacon, and place in slow cooker.
4. Cook chicken breast on high for 4 hours.

5. Place mayonnaise with 1 tsp black pepper and 4 tbsp extra virgin olive oil in blender. Mix until smooth.
6. Combine lettuce, tomato in bowl, and toss with mayo dressing.
7. Top salad with chicken breast and serve.

Nutrition per serving:

Calories 366

Carbs 6 g

Fat 19 g

Protein 43 g

Sodium 1183 mg

Sugar 0 g

Figs and Goat Cheese-Stuffed Chicken

Serves: 4

Preparation time: 20 minutes

Cooking time: 8 hours

Ingredients:

4 x 4oz chicken breasts

4 figs

½ cup goat cheese, crumbled

1 tsp salt

1 tsp black pepper

Extra virgin olive oil

Directions:

1. Combine 3 tbsp olive oil, salt, black pepper in bowl, and rub onto chicken breasts. Marinate for an hour.
2. Remove fig skin, and slice figs into ½" pieces. Combine with goat cheese.
3. Turn slow cooker to low.
4. Place plastic wrap over chicken breasts and pound with mallet until each breast is approximately ¼" thick (or ask your butcher to do it).

5. Scoop a quarter of the cheese-fig mixture into chicken, roll up chicken breast and place in slow cooker.
6. Repeat for each chicken breast.
7. Cook on low for 8 hours.
8. Serve with a green salad.

Nutrition per serving:

Calories 369

Carbs 7 g

Fat 18 g

Protein 46 g

Sodium 811 mg

Sugar 0 g

Carne Asada

Serves: 8

Preparation Time: 10 minutes

Cooking Time: 8 hours

Ingredients:

4 lb chuck roast

1 onion, chopped

4 limes, juiced

½ cup cilantro, minced

8 cloves garlic, minced

2 tsp paprika

2 tsp oregano

2 tsp cumin

2 tsp salt

1 tsp black pepper

Directions:

1. Rinse pot roast and pat dry.
2. Combine remaining ingredients in blender, and mix until well combined.
3. Brush slow cooker with extra virgin olive oil, and set on high.
4. Coat pot roast with cilantro topping.
5. Place in slow cooker, and cook for 8 hours.
6. Serve with Cauliflower Rice.

Nutrition per serving:

Calories 506

Carbs 3 g

Fat 19 g

Protein 75 g

Sodium 733 mg

Sugar 0 g

Amazing Pulled Pork

Serves: 8

Preparation Time: 25 minutes

Cooking Time: 8 hours

Ingredients:

5 lb pork shoulder

2 tbsp mustard

2 cups tomato purée

6 Medjool Dates, pitted

½ tsp cloves, ground

½ tsp cinnamon

2 tsp salt

Extra virgin olive oil

Tortilla Wraps

8 eggs

1 tbsp coconut flour

½ tsp salt

Directions:

1. Place pitted dates in blender, and mix until paste forms, add tomato purée, cinnamon, salt, black pepper, and mix.

2. Combine mustard, blended tomato puree, cloves, cinnamon, salt, and mix.
3. Place pork shoulder in slow cooker, pour sauce into slow cooker, and coat pork shoulder.
4. Cook pork for 8 hours on high.
5. Once pork is cooked, use fork to shred.
6. For tortilla wraps, whisk eggs, add milk and flour, and mix until well combined.
7. Heat 4 tbsp oil in skillet on medium-high.
8. Pour 1/8th of mixture into skillet and cook each side 30 seconds.
9. Spoon pork mixture into egg tortilla and serve.

Nutrition per serving:

Calories 777

Carbs 8 g

Fat 55 g

Protein 59 g

Sodium 835 mg

Sugar 5 g

Braised Pork Belly

Serves: 8

Preparation Time: 10 minutes

Cooking Time: 4 hours

Ingredients:

1 lb pork belly

2 medium onions, diced

1 tsp Dijon mustard

½ cup apple sauce

1 tsp black pepper

1 tsp salt

Directions:

1. Heat extra virgin olive oil in skillet, add onion, sauté for a minute.
2. Place onion in slow cooker, add pork belly, apple sauce. Cook on high for 4 hours.
3. Serve with Walnut Cabbage Salad.

Nutrition per serving:

Calories 278

Carbs 3.5 g

Fat 15 g

Protein 26 g

Sodium 1214 mg

Sugar 2 g

Peppercorn Short Ribs

Serves: 8

Preparation Time: 10 minutes

Cooking Time: 4 hours

Ingredients:

4 lbs short ribs, bone in

8 peppercorns

2 cups low-sodium beef

1 onion, diced

2 carrots, peeled, diced

2 celery stalks, diced

4 cloves, minced

1 tsp thyme

1 tsp rosemary

2 bay leaves

2 tsp salt

2 tsp black pepper

Extra virgin olive oil

Directions:

1. Heat 4 tbsp extra virgin olive oil in skillet. Add onions and garlic, and sauté until brown.
2. Place onion mixture in slow cooker, add short ribs along with carrots, celery stalk, cloves, thyme,

rosemary, peppercorns, bay leaves, salt, and black pepper.

3. Cook on high for 4 hours.

Nutrition per serving:

Calories 520

Carbs 3.7 g

Fat 24 g

Protein 67 g

Sodium 923 mg

Sugar 0 g

Spicy Italian Sausage and Zucchini Noodles

Serves: 6

Preparation Time: 20 minutes

Cooking Time: 4 hours

Ingredients

6 Spicy Italian pork sausages

1 onion, peeled and diced

2 cups low-sodium chicken stock

1 tomato, diced

4 zucchinis, peeled

1 tsp oregano

1 tsp salt

1 tsp black pepper

Extra virgin olive oil

Directions

1. Coat slow cooker with a little extra virgin olive oil, and set to high.
2. Slice sausage into ½" thick rounds, and place in slow cooker.
3. Heat 3 tbsp extra virgin olive oil in skillet, add onion and garlic, sauté for a minute, and add to slow cooker.

4. Add tomatoes, oregano, and a tsp of salt and black pepper along with chicken stock, cover and cook for 4 hours.
5. Using Mandolin, slice zucchini vertically to create thin Zucchini Noodles.
6. Top zucchini noodles with Spicy Italian Sausage and serve.

Nutrition per serving:

Calories 254

Carbs 8.5 g

Fat 14 g

Protein 24 g

Sodium 1044 mg

Sugar 3 g

Meaty Cauliflower Lasagna

Serves: 8

Preparation Time: 20 minutes

Cooking Time: 5 hours

Ingredients:

1 lb ground beef

1 small cauliflower head

1 red onion, diced

4 cloves garlic, minced

2 cups crushed tomato

1 cup Mozzarella, shredded

1 egg

1 tsp oregano

1 bay leaf

1 tsp black pepper

1 tsp salt

Extra virgin olive oil

Directions:

1. Brush slow cooker with olive oil, and set slow cooker on medium high.
2. Separate cauliflower into florets, peel outer layer of cauliflower stem, and dice stem.

3. Place cauliflower in food processor, and pulse into rice-like granules, crack an egg into cauliflower, and mix along with ½ tsp of salt.
4. Place 3 tbsp olive oil in skillet, add ground beef, brown, add crushed tomatoes, oregano, bay leaf, black pepper and ½ tsp salt, mix.
5. Place ½ cauliflower mixture in slow cooker, next layer ⅓of beef mixture and ½ of cheese, place remaining cauliflower on top. Spoon remaining sauce on top of cauliflower, sprinkle with remaining cheese.
6. Cook on medium high for 5 hours.

Nutrition per serving:

Calories 342

Carbs 8.2 g

Fat 14 g

Protein 45 g

Sodium 681 mg

Sugar 0 g

Chili Verde

Serves: 8

Preparation Time: 10 minutes

Cooking Time: 7 hours

Ingredients:

1½ lbs pork shoulder

½ lb sirloin, cubed

4 Anaheim chilies, stemmed

6 cloves garlic, minced

½ cup cilantro, chopped

2 onions, peeled and sliced

2 tomatoes, chopped.

1 tbsp tomato paste

1 lime

1 tbsp cumin

1 tbsp oregano

Extra virgin olive oil

Directions:

1. Slice pork shoulder into ½" cubes, and set slow cooker to medium.
2. Heat 4 tbsp extra virgin olive oil in skillet, add onions, Anaheim chilies, and garlic, and sauté for 2 minutes.

3. Place skillet mixture into slow cooker, add pork shoulder, sirloin, and stir.
4. Add tomatoes, cilantro, tomato paste, cumin, oregano, and salt to pot.
5. Cover and cook for 7 hours.
6. Squeeze a little of lime in each bowl when serving.

Nutrition per serving:

Calories 262

Carbs 6 g

Fat 16 g

Protein 23 g

Sodium 63 mg

Sugar 0 g

Tandoori Salmon with Fresh Cucumber Salad

Serves: 8

Preparation Time: 10 minutes

Cooking Time: 3 hours

Ingredients:

4 x 4oz Wild salmon fillets

2 tsp Tandoori spice

1 tsp salt

1 tsp black pepper

4 tbsp ghee

Cucumber Salad

1 English cucumber

1 cup arugula

½ cup parsley

¼ cup lemon juice

2 tbsp extra virgin olive oil

Directions:

1. Heat ghee in skillet over medium heat along with tandoori spice for a minute.

2. Place salmon filets in slow cooker, skin side down, sprinkle with salt, black pepper, and pour Tandoori butter over salmon.
3. Cook on high for 3.5 hours.
4. While salmon is cooking, dice cucumber, and toss with arugula, parsley, lemon juice and extra virgin olive oil.
5. Serve salmon with fresh cucumber salad.

Nutrition per serving:

Calories 413

Carbs 4 g

Fat 34 g

Protein 25 g

Sodium 645 mg

Sugar 0 g

CONCLUSION

It is absolutely essential to know exactly what you are putting into your body when you commit to living the ketogenic lifestyle, and sometimes that can seem a little overwhelming. The Ketogenic Slow Cooker Recipes cookbook has been designed with you in mind. That is why these recipes have been created to ensure that you are worry-free when you whip up any of the dishes in this book.

All of the nutrients have been calculated so that your body can remain in ketosis. Beyond the technicalities, you can also rest assured that all of your meals will be delicious and nutritious. By the way, slow cooking also helps to inject extra rich layers of flavor into just about any dish, and the wonderful scents wafting through your home don't hurt either.

We hope the Ketogenic Slow Cooker Recipes cookbook serves as an easy go-to source for all of your cooking needs so that you can enjoy all of the benefits of the ketogenic lifestyle without any of the fuss.

APPENDIX

Cooking Conversion Charts

1. Volumes

US Fluid Oz.	US	US Dry Oz.	Metric Liquid ml
¼ oz.	2 tsp.	1 oz.	10 ml.
½ oz.	1 tbsp.	2 oz.	15 ml.
1 oz.	2 tbsp.	3 oz.	30 ml.
2 oz.	¼ cup	3½ oz.	60 ml.
4 oz.	½ cup	4 oz.	125 ml.
6 oz.	¾ cup	6 oz.	175 ml.
8 oz.	1 cup	8 oz.	250 ml.

Tsp.= teaspoon - tbsp.= tablespoon – oz.= ounce – ml.= millimeter

2. Oven Temperatures

Celsius (ºC)	Fahrenheit (ºF)
90	220
110	225
120	250
140	275
150	300
160	325
180	350
190	375
200	400
215	425
230	450
250	475
260	500

Made in the USA
San Bernardino, CA
04 November 2016